I0053915

Making Penicillin

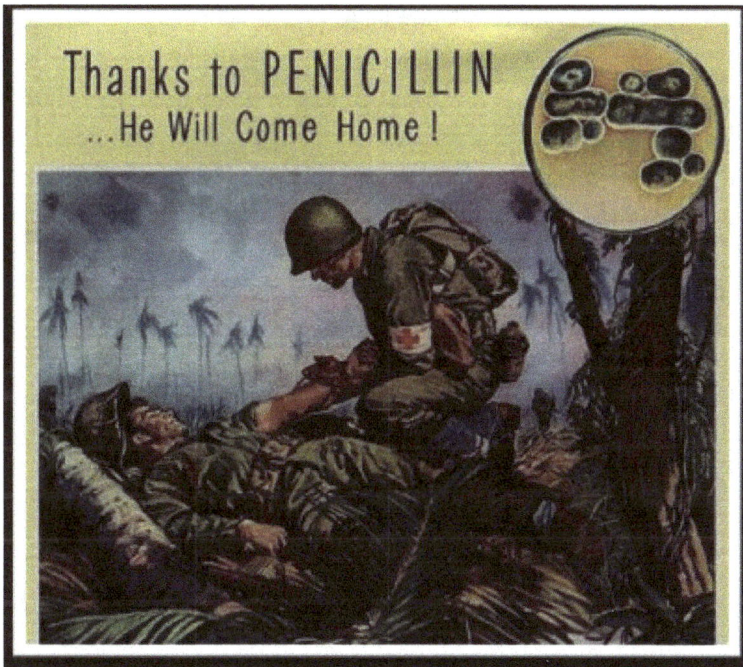

Thanks to PENICILLIN
...He Will Come Home!

WHO

Copyright

Reference Study Guide

Survival Antibiotics:

Will Your Demise Be A Sinus Infection?

Thanks to PENICILLIN
...He Will Come Home!

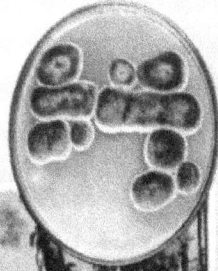

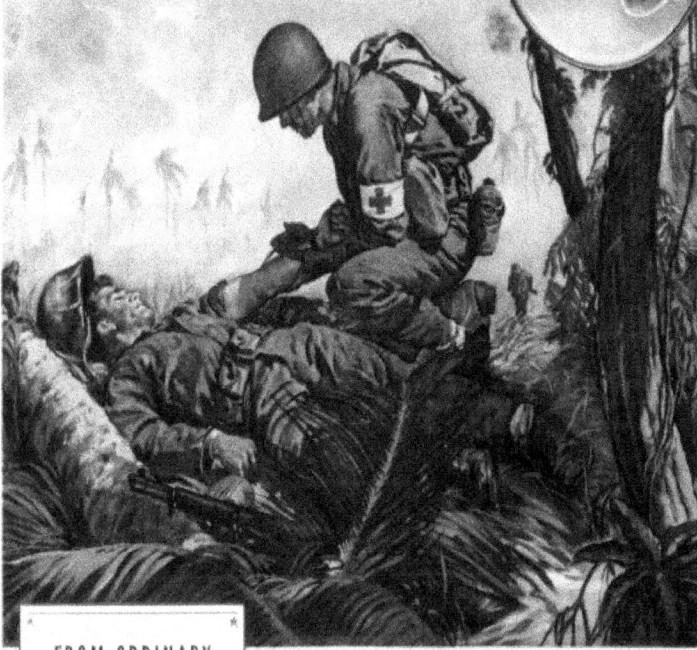

FROM ORDINARY MOLD—
the Greatest Healing Agent of this War!

On the gauzy, green-and-yellow mold above, called *Penicillium notatum* in the laboratory, grows the miraculous substance first discovered by Professor Alexander Fleming in 1928. Named penicillin by its discoverer, it is the most potent weapon ever developed against many of the deadliest infections known to man. Because research on molds was already a part of Schenley enterprise, Schenley Laboratories were well able to meet the problem of large-scale production of penicillin, when the great need for it arose.

When the thunderous battles of this war have subsided to pages of silent print in a history book, the greatest news event of World War II may well be the discovery and development — not of some vicious secret weapon that *destroys* — but of a weapon that *saves* lives. That weapon, of course, is penicillin.

Every day, penicillin is performing some unbelievable act of healing on some far battlefront. Thousands of men will return home who otherwise would not have had a chance. Better still, more and more of this precious drug is now available for civilian use ... to save the lives of persons of every age.

A year ago, production of penicillin was difficult, costly. Today, due to specially-devised methods of mass-production, in use by Schenley Laboratories, Inc. and the 20 other firms designated by the government to make penicillin, it is available in ever-increasing quantity, at progressively lower cost.

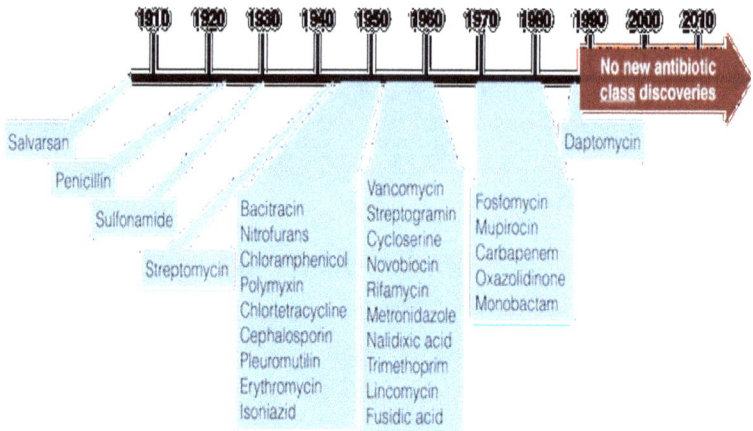

Timeline of antibiotic discovery

Year	Antibiotics
1910	Salvarsan
1920	Penicillin
1930	Sulfonamide
1940	Streptomycin
1950	Bacitracin, Nitrofurans, Chloramphenicol, Polymyxin, Chlortetracycline, Cephalosporin, Pleuromutilin, Erythromycin, Isoniazid
1960	Vancomycin, Streptogramin, Cycloserine, Novobiocin, Rifamycin, Metronidazole, Nalidixic acid, Trimethoprim, Lincomycin, Fusidic acid
1970	Fosfomycin, Mupirocin, Carbapenem, Oxazolidinone, Monobactam
1980	
1990	Daptomycin
2000	No new antibiotic class discoveries
2010	

4

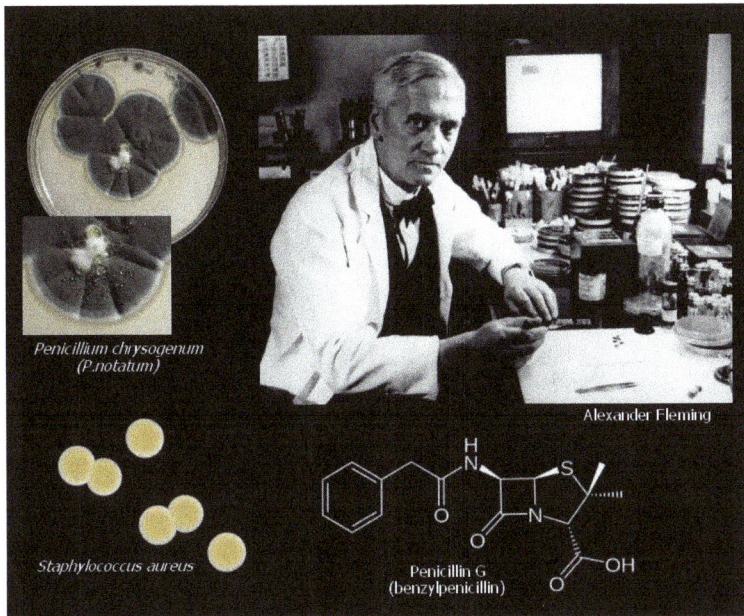

Penicillium chrysogenum
(P.notatum)

Alexander Fleming

Staphylococcus aureus

Penicillin G
(benzylpenicillin)

World War II saw major advances in medical technology including the mass production of penicillin. On March 15, 1942, U.S. made-penicillin was used to successfully treat the first patient for septicemia, blood poisoning. This one treatment alone exhausted half of the available supply of penicillin in the

United States, so the need for better techniques for produce penicillin rapidly on a large scale was necessary to help treat and U.S. soldiers fighting in Europe.

Scientists working around the clock manufactured 2.4 million doses of penicillin in preparation for the D-Day landings alone, on June 6, 1944.

Discovery

Sir Alexander Fleming discovered the bacteria-killing properties of penicillin while conducting research at St. Mary's Hospital in London in the late 1920s. Upon returning to his disorganized lab from a weekend vacation, Fleming noticed that one of the Petri dishes was uncovered and a blue-green mold was growing inside. Rather than tossing the contaminated dish into the trash, he looked carefully and observed that the mold had killed bacteria growing nearby. Quite by accident Fleming had discovered penicillin, the antibiotic released by the mold of the genus Penicillium.

Alexander Fleming was familiar with the treatment of bacterial infections after spending World

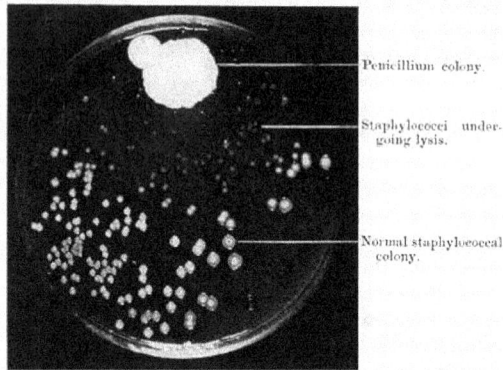

Fleming's original photograph of the contaminated dish.

In War I as a captain in the British Medical Corps. Fleming saw firsthand the lack of medicine to treat infections, with disease causing approximately one third of military deaths during the Great War.

Despite its historical significance, Fleming's discovery of penicillin in 1928 brought little attention. The technology and funding needed to isolate and produce the antibiotic was unavailable at the time. Fleming, however, continued to grow the Penicillium notatum strain in his lab for twelve years, distributing it to scientists and saving the specimen for someone willing and able to transform the "mold juice" into a medicine suitable for human use.

Purification and Trials

Meanwhile, Australian scientist Howard Florey hired Ernst Chain to help with his microbiology research at

Oxford University. Florey and Chain were interested in Alexander Fleming's work and in 1938, began studying the antibacterial properties of mold. Chain began by purifying and concentrating the penicillin "juice" through a complex and tiring process of freeze drying the product repeatedly. This slow and relatively inefficient process was improved upon by another researcher, Norman Heatley, who purified the penicillin by adjusting the acidity, or pH.

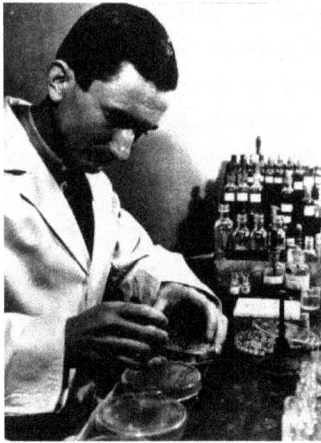

Norman Heatley working with Penicillium cultures. Photograph William Dunn School of Pathology, University of Oxford.

To their great excitement, Florey's team successfully cured infected mice with penicillin on May 25, 1940. Heatley oversaw the trials and recorded in his diary, "After supper with some friends, I returned to the lab and met the professor to give a final dose of penicillin to two of the mice.

The 'controls' were looking very sick, but the two treated mice seemed very well. I stayed at the lab until 3:45am, by which time all four control animals were dead." Delirious with excitement, Heatley returned home early that morning, surprised to find that he had put his underpants on backwards in the dark! The usually mild-mannered Heatley noted in his journal, "It really looks as if penicillin may be of practical importance."

Mass Production

Florey and Chain's report about the mouse trials drew great interest from both scientific and military communities.

World War II was well underway in Europe and the ability to combat disease and infection could mean the difference between victory and defeat. Because British facilities were manufacturing other drugs needed for the war effort in Europe, Florey and Heatley travelled to the U.S. in July of 1941 to continue research and seek help from the American pharmaceutical industry. They convinced four drug companies, Merck, E. R. Squibb & Sons, Charles Pfizer & Co., and Lederle Laboratories, to aid in the production of penicillin.

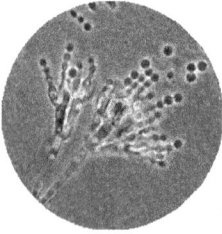
Penicillium notatum viewed with a microscope, 400x.

Florey and Heatley ended up in Peoria, Illinois to work with researchers who had perfected the fermentation process necessary for growing penicillin. The researchers in Peoria used corn instead of glucose, or simple sugar, as the nutrient source, and the penicillin grew approximately 500 times more than it had in England!

The team searched for more productive strains of Penicillium notatum, finding the best specimen growing on an over-ripe cantaloupe in a Peoria grocery store.

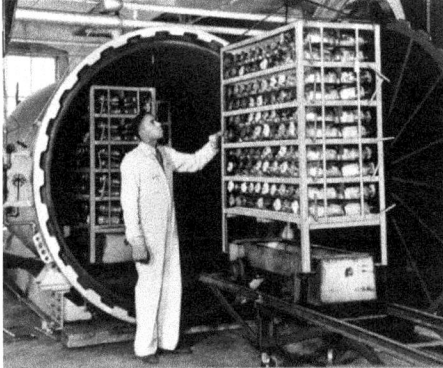

Penicillin production at pharmaceutical company, Eli Lilly.

Meanwhile, penicillin was used to cure the first human bacterial infection, proving to researchers the vital importance of the drug to save lives. But, that one cure used up the entire supply of penicillin in the entire U.S! Following Japan's attack on Pearl Harbor on December 7, 1941, it was clear to scientists and military strategists that a combined effort was needed to produce the large amounts of penicillin needed to win the war. A total of 21 U.S. companies joined together, producing 2.3 million doses of penicillin in preparation of the D-Day invasion of Normandy. Penicillin quickly became known as the war's "miracle drug," curing infectious disease and saving millions of lives.

In 1945, Sir Alexander Fleming, Ernst Chain, Sir Howard Florey were awarded the Nobel Prize in Physiology or Medicine "for the discovery of penicillin and its curative effect in various infectious diseases." We have modern antibiotics today because scientists and drug companies worked together to solve a problem.

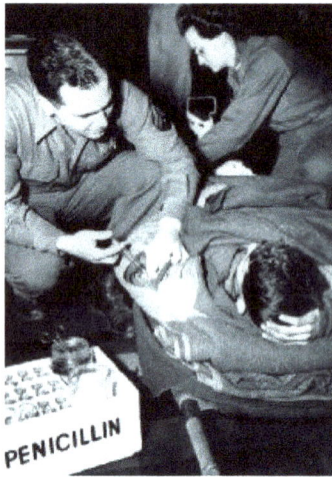

Medics using penicillin to combat infections in soldiers

Infection is always a killer, and while some soap and water could prevent it externally, but when the infection becomes inside humans, then we are often very helpless. And most anti-bacterial agent injected into the body would kill a human more quickly than the infection would.

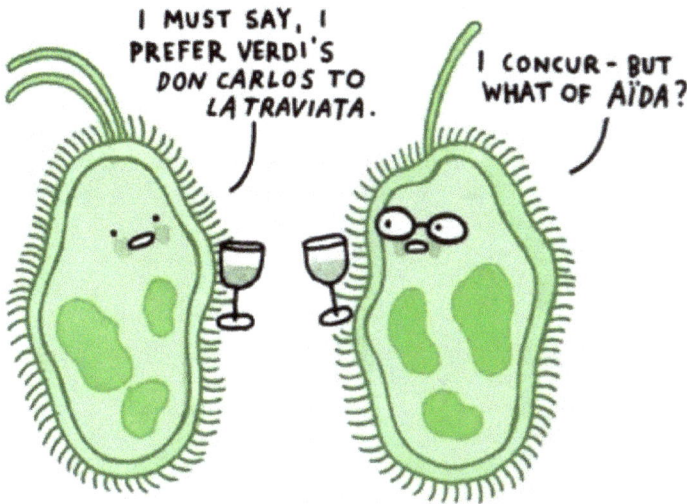

CULTURED BACTERIA

FOR MANY YEARS, scientists knew that certain molds killed some bacteria. However, researchers needed to understand how to harness this antibacterial microbe and to manufacture enough of the substance before they could make a useful medicine.

(1) *Penicillium* mold naturally produces the antibiotic penicillin

(2) Scientists learned to grow *Penicillium* mold in deep fermentation tanks by adding a kind of sugar and other ingredients. This process increased the growth of *Penicillium*.

(3) Then, scientists separated the penicillin product from the mold.

(4) Finally, penicillin is purified for use as an antibiotic medicine.

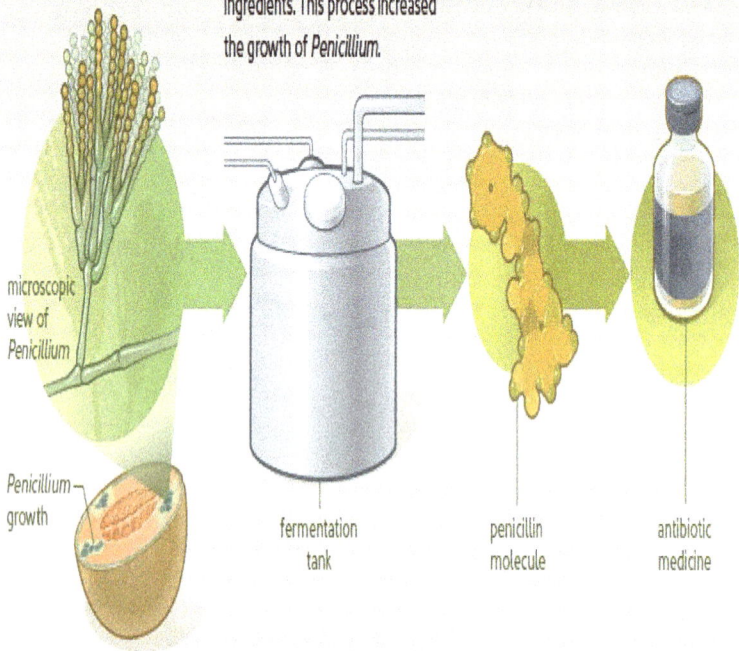

microscopic view of *Penicillium*

Penicillium growth

fermentation tank

penicillin molecule

antibiotic medicine

The rest of the book shows you how to make Penicillin Correctly with a simple Formula.

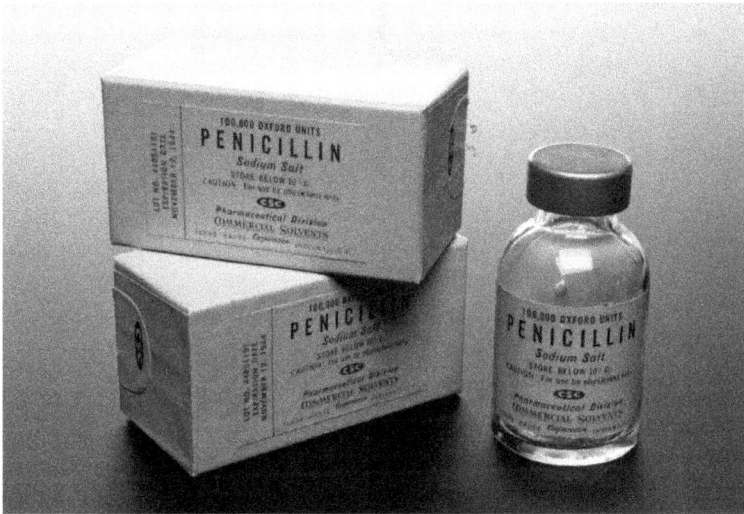

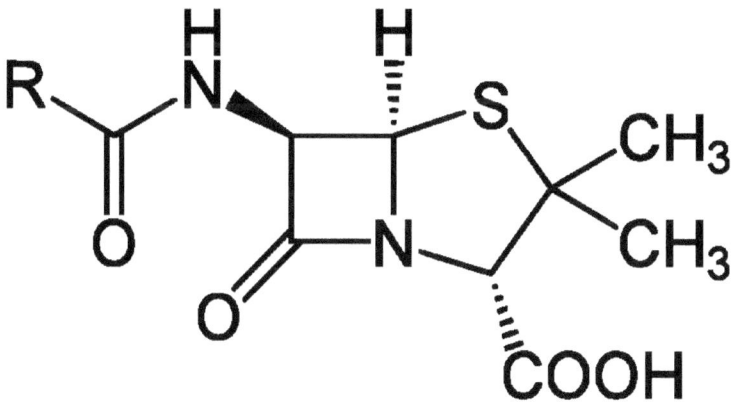

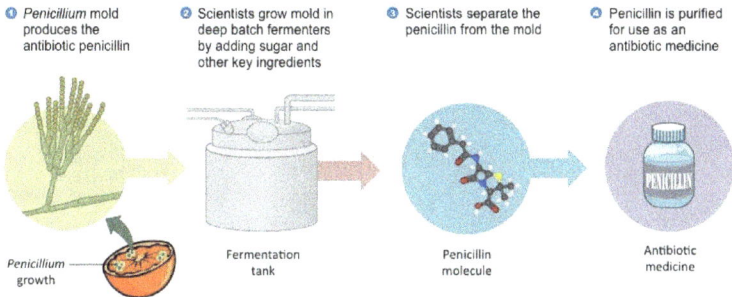

1 *Penicillium* mold produces the antibiotic penicillin

2 Scientists grow mold in deep batch fermenters by adding sugar and other key ingredients

3 Scientists separate the penicillin from the mold

4 Penicillin is purified for use as an antibiotic medicine

Penicillium growth

Fermentation tank

Penicillin molecule

Antibiotic medicine

Penicillin is an antibiotic that is used to fight pathogenic bacteria in the human body. Penicillin was truly the beginning of the antibiotic age. It was discovered in 1928, by the researcher Alexander Fleming. He figured out that bacteria in a simple petri dish that was full of Staphylococcus colonies could not grow in the mold.

However, after Alexander Fleming isolated the source from the mold, the medical world was changed for the better.

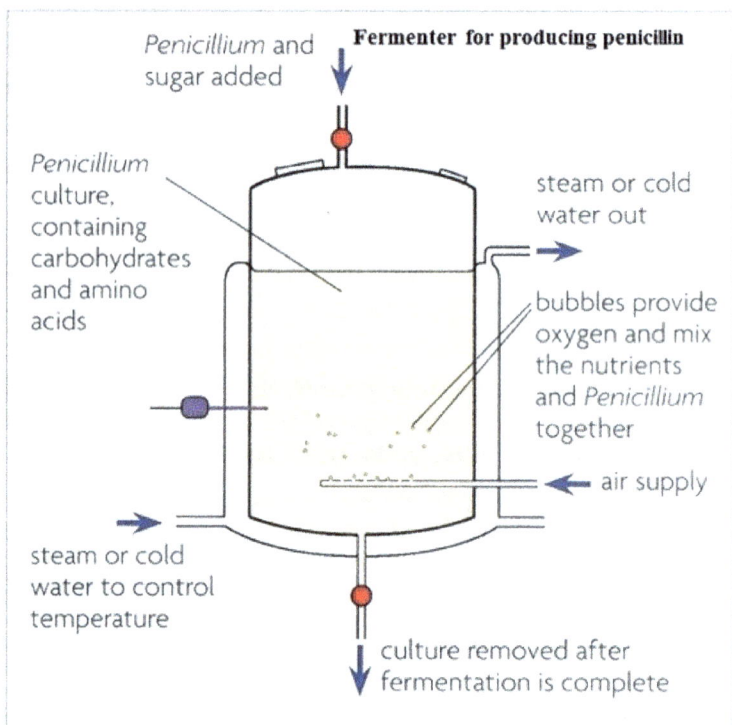

Fermenter for producing penicillin

Penicillium and sugar added

Penicillium culture, containing carbohydrates and amino acids

steam or cold water out

bubbles provide oxygen and mix the nutrients and *Penicillium* together

air supply

steam or cold water to control temperature

culture removed after fermentation is complete

Because of Alexander Fleming, doctors w0ere able to treat conditions such as pneumonia and rheumatic fever.

Pneumonia and rheumatic fever killed millions of people because of the lack of medical supplies that were affective.

Penicillin is a simply a byproduct of the Penicillium fungus. Believe it or not, you can make it at home. But you should not attempt to make your own penicillin. Because if you have access to a hospital, then leave it to the professionals make Penicillin. The information in this book is purely for illustrative purposes, such as if you are stuck on Mars where it is impossible to access antibiotics.

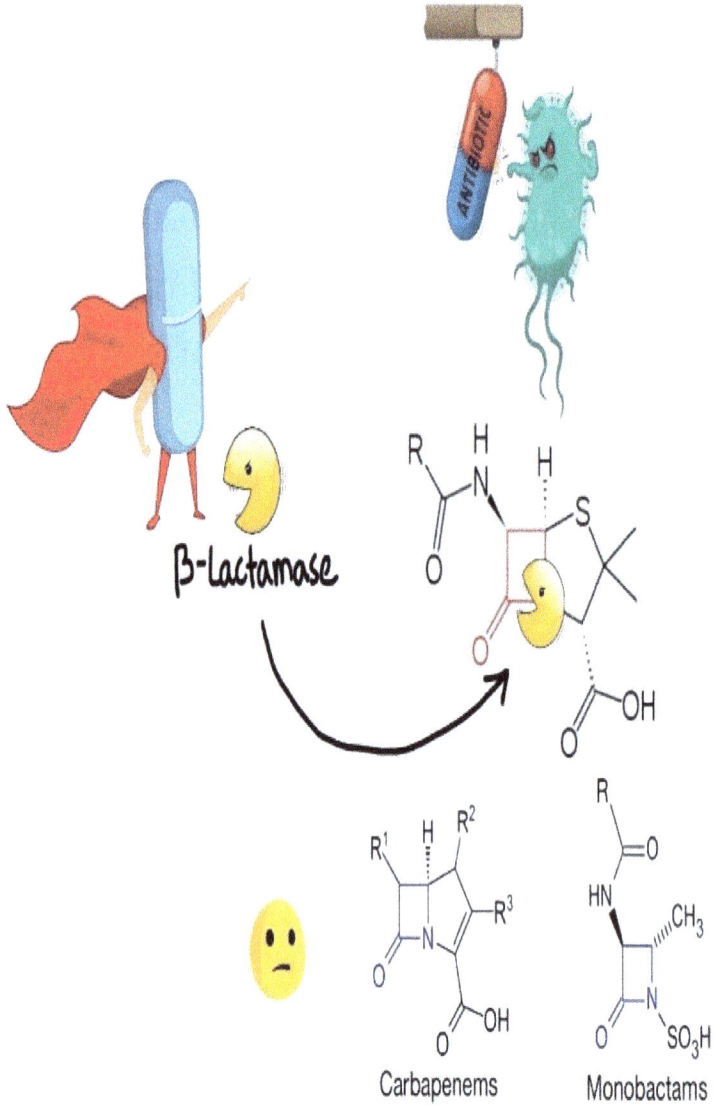

β-Lactamase

Carbapenems

Monobactams

THE FORMULA FOR PENICILLIN

Penicillin mold

Penicillium Notatum mold

As we stated before, Penicillin is a by-product of the Penicillium fungus. It is a by-product of a Penicillium fungus that is under stress.

First you have to grow the fungus, and then expose it to stresses to make it produce Penicillin.

First you need to produce a **culture** of the penicillium fungus.

A microbiological culture is simply a way of reproducing a microscopic organism by letting them reproduce in a certain environment under controlled conditions.

STEP 1

First try to expose a slice of bread or citrus peel or even a cantaloupe rind to the air in a very dark place at 70 degrees F, until a bluish-green mold develops.

Now cut two fresh slices of whole wheat bread into ½ inch cubes. Place the cubes in a 750 ml Erlenmeyer flask with a non-absorbent plug.

Note: A lot of bakeries put a substance called a mold inhibitor on their bread. This mold inhibitor will suppress fungal growth. Therefore, you must use bread that you baked yourself.

Now you must sterilize the flask and its contents in a pressure cooker for at least 20 minutes at 15 psi.

Another, method is to place it in an oven at 315 degrees Fahrenheit for one hour.

In a sterile fashion, now you must transfer the fungus from the bread or fruit peel into our flask that has our bread cubes.

Now allow the cubes to sit in a very dark place at 70 degrees F for about 5 days. This is what we call incubation. This is the easy part.

STEP 2

Now here is where it gets very complicated. You must prepare one liter of the following liquid solution:

Lactose Monohydrate	44.0 gm
Corn Starch	25.0 gm
Sodium Nitrate	3.0 gm
Magnesium Sulfate	0.25 gm
Potassium MonoPhosphate	0.50 gm
Glucose Monohydrate	2.75 gm
Zinc Sulfate	0.044 gm
Manganese Sulfate	0.044 gm

The above simple ingredients can always be found at many chemical supply houses, but you have to buy a significant amount.

Now dissolve all the ingredients in the order listed above in 500ml of cold tap water. Once you are done, then add more cold water to complete a liter (1000 ml).

After you have added the water, you must adjust the pH to 5.0-5.5 using HCL (hydrochloric acid). Here, you will need a simple pH test kit. You can find at a pet shop or most garden supply stores.

Next, you must fill glass containers with a quantity of this solution. Make sure that you use enough so that when the container is placed on its side our liquid will not touch the plug.

Next sterilize the containers and the solution in a pressure cooker or stove as we did before. Now when it cools, scrape up approximately a tablespoon of the fungus from our bread cubes and throw it into the solution.

Now you must allow the containers to incubate on their sides at 70 degrees F for about seven days.

It is very important that they are not moved around. Now if you did it correctly, you will have Penicillin in the liquid portion of the media.

Now simply filter the mixture through a coffee filter, or a thin cloth, or something similar, then plug the bottle containers, and refrigerate them immediately.

STEP 3

How to extract our penicillin from the solution:

Simply adjust the cold solution to pH 2.2 using (.01 %) HCL. Then mix it with cold ethyl acetate in a **separatory funnel** (this is a funnel with a stopcock, you can find most or all these items at chemistry glass suppliers) and shake well for about 30 seconds or so.

Now drain the ethyl acetate, which is on the bottom, into a clean beaker which has been placed in an ice bath and repeat the process.

Now add 1% potassium acetate and mix well. We want the ethyl acetate to evaporate off.

This can be done or induced by a constant flow of air over the top of the beaker, like from a fan. Wait until it dries. The remaining crystals are simply a mixture of potassium penicillin and potassium acetate.

That is it! You just built a simple laboratory and made you have truly made Penicillin!

Now you are the mad scientist that just made Penicillin!

Foods that Fights Respiratory and Fungal Infections

Fungal infections forms: *candida, athletes foot, yeast infection.* Starving the yeast is the best way to treat fungal infections.

Fungi are primitive organisms and are everywhere in our environment such as in our air, in the soil, even on plants and in water. We see Fungi almost every day, such as mildew, mold. Mushrooms are a form of fungi too.

In the woman's vagina, a candida infection is commonly known as a yeast infection.

People with diabetes get yeast infections often. Vinegar and Apple cider vinegar are a scientifically proven antifungal. Laboratory research shows that it can inhibit the growth of candida cultivating in a petri dish.

I also recommend adding a tea spoon of Apple Cider to your bird's or parrot's water dish. And like humans, cats and dogs do not like vinegar much, but it is good for them. Add a spoon of Apple Cider each day to their fresh water bowl. Add Apple Cider only once a day, but change the water bowl twice a day, so pets that are sensitive to vinegar are not harmed.

If fungi and yeast is everywhere, then why humans are not sick all the time? This is because only half of all types of fungi are very harmful, but the other half is perfectly benign. While oral antifungal and topical medications are often necessary, the food we eat can often prevent or treat fungal infections. Many plant and foods have fungal fighting properties such as anti-parasitic, anti-microbial, and anti-bacterial agents.

Foods that have high fungal fighting properties include:

- Vinegar
- Apple cider vinegar
- Garlic
- Onion
- Coconut oil
- Ginger
- Pumpkin seeds
- Cinnamon, cloves
- Lemons and Lime

Next I will present many food recipes that will incorporate these all the natural fungus-fighting foods.

1. Crispy Rice with Coconut Oil

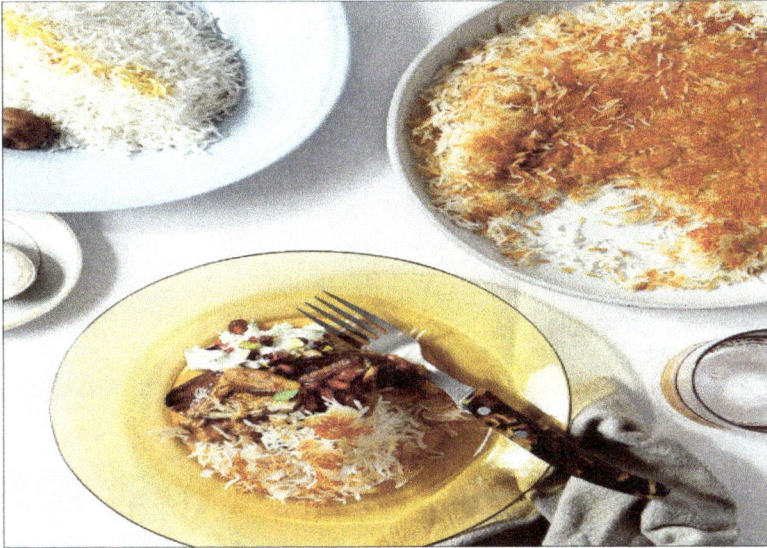

Coconut Oil and products fights off fungal infections. Coconut oil has strong antifungal and antibacterial properties. It fights off fungal infections such as yeast and candida infections. This Crispy Rice with Coconut Oil dish uses 3 tablespoons of fungus fighting coconut oil.

2. Muffins with Apple Cider

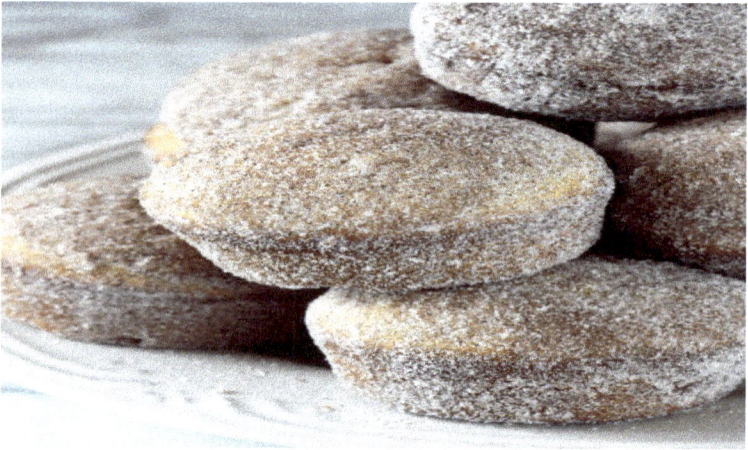

Apple cider vinegar which is made from crushed, aged, and fermented apples is great for all sorts of cuisines and due to its colonies of good bacteria, it can also be used as a body cleanser. Apple cider vinegar is a strong and effective fungus killer. These Muffins with Apple Cider has 1/3 cup of apple cider vinegar, combined with fungus fighting cinnamon. Use coconut oil instead of canola oil and you have a powerful fungus fighting treat.

3. Blistered Shishitos with Ginger plus Garlic

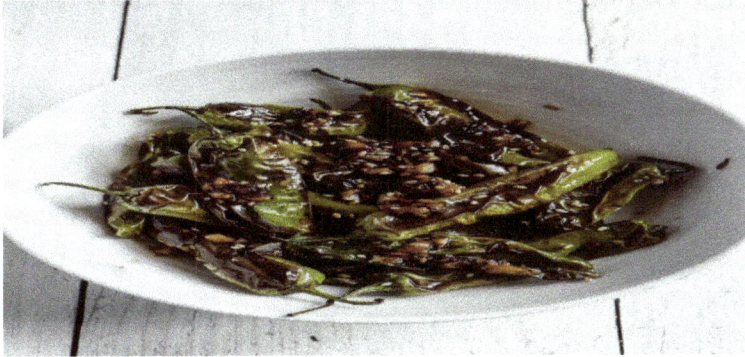

Ginger and garlic have strong antibacterial and antifungal properties. Ginger and garlic have been used since Jesus's time as natural remedies for many ailments. Allicin is a compound produced when garlic is crushed or chopped. It has a very potent antibiotic quality. Ginger which is often used to treat nausea, also has antifungal properties. These Blistered Shishito Peppers with Ginger and Garlic are easy to make and can make a wonderful treat. Along with the garlic cloves and minced ginger, add fresh lime juice and healthy olive oil and fat-filled sesame.

4. Coconut Kaffir Lime Cooler

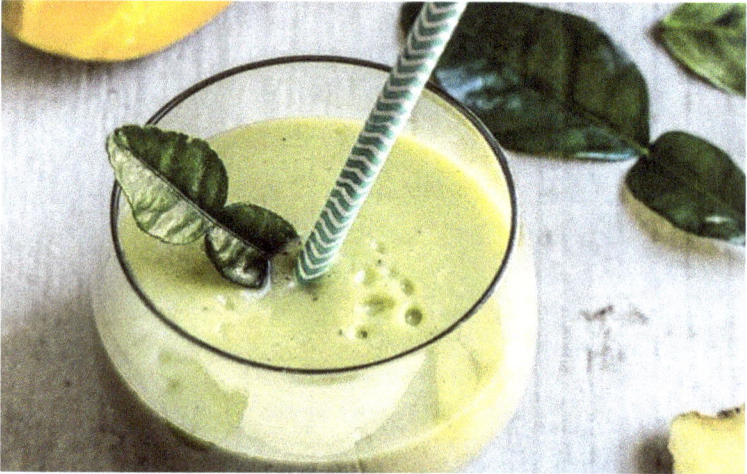

Packing a powerful antifungal one-two punch, this Coconut Kaffir Lime Cooler calls for two coconut-rich products — milk and water — along with a dose of fresh antifungal and antibacterial ginger. This beverage infuses the nutrients together with a bit of citrus and the sweet tang of fresh mango!

5. Garlic Miso and Onion Soup

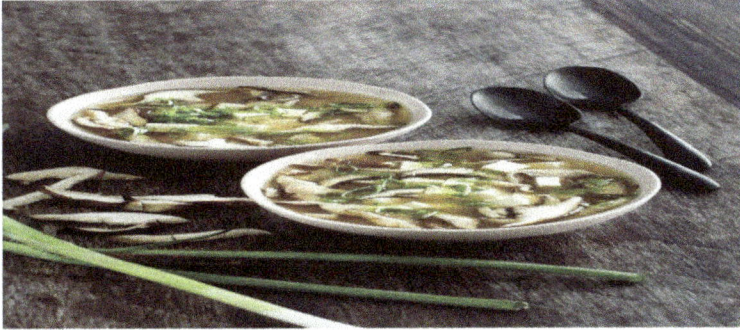

Onions are not only an aromatic pleasure and flavor enhancer, but they also have antifungal, antibacterial, and antiparasitic properties. Plus, onions also "help the kidneys to flush excess fluids out the body," keeping sodium and water levels balanced in the body. This Garlic Miso and Onion Soup calls for one and a half onions, four whole cloves of garlic, and a half of a cup of shiitake mushrooms, all of which are great for fighting fungal infections. In addition, this soup uses protein-rich tofu, fermented miso and soy sauce, and healthy fat-filled sesame oil.

6. Homemade Pumpkin Seed Milk

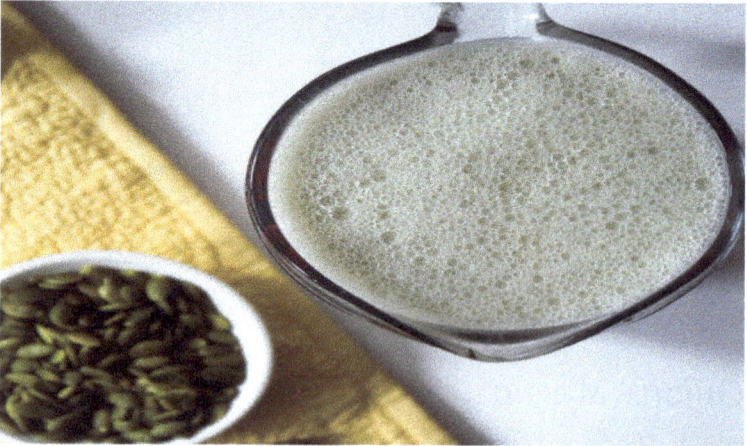

Seeds are a staple in any plant-based diet as they are usually high in fat and other essential nutrients. Pumpkin seeds are no exception! They are high in omega-3 fatty acids, plus these tasty seeds "have antifungal, antiviral and anti-parasitic properties." This Homemade Pumpkin Seed Milk is a rich and tasty source of pumpkin seeds! The recipe calls for a full cup of pumpkin seeds and adds a warming flavor with nutmeg, dates, and vanilla extract.

7. Rhubarb and Ginger Shrub Drinking Vinegar

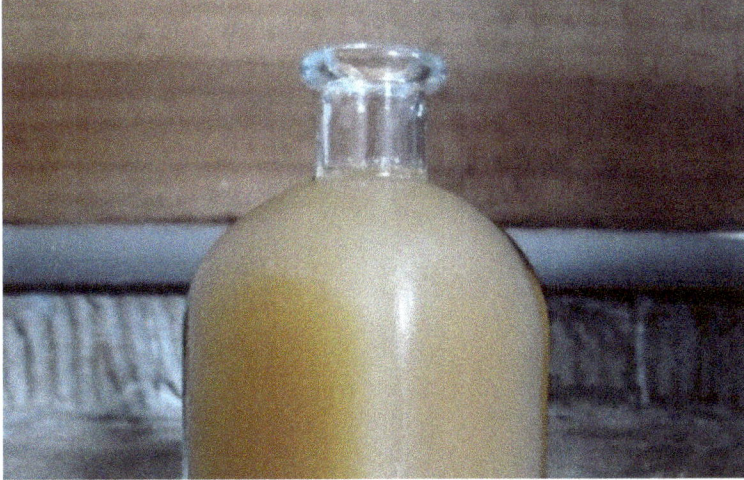

While apple cider vinegar is excellent for baking sweet treats, it can also be used to give beverages a spicy-sweet kick of flavor! This Rhubarb and Ginger Shrub Drinking Vinegar calls for fungus-fighting a full cup of apple cider vinegar and two tablespoons of fresh ginger.

8. Cinnamon and Clove Mixed Nut and Seed Milk

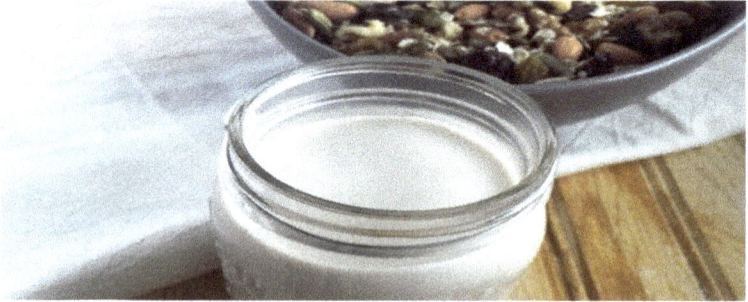

Cinnamon and cloves offer two ends of the spice spectrum — one being warm, spicy, and sweet, while the other is earthy, nutty, and rich. As different as their flavors are, both of these spices are great for fighting fungal infections. Cinnamon "has been used as an anti-inflammatory and anticancer agent," while cloves have a variety of antifungal and immune system stimulating constituents. This Cinnamon and Clove Mixed Nut and Seed Milk calls for both cinnamon and cloves, along with a host of nutrient-dense nuts and seeds.

9. Cinnamon Linseed Pancakes

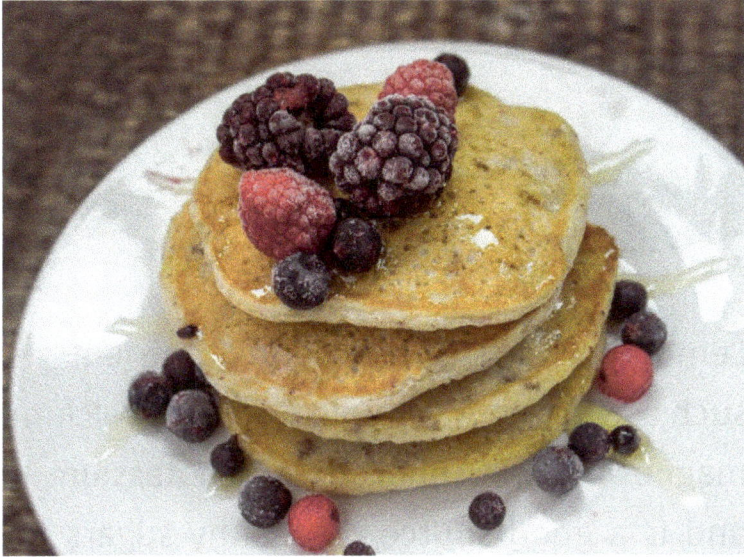

Looking for a warm and tasty recipe to get your body going in the morning? These Cinnamon Linseed Pancakes not only will boost your digestion for the day with a helping of fiber-rich linseed (also known as flaxseed), but it also uses fungus-fighting cinnamon and coconut oil!

10. Lemon Sautéed Asparagus

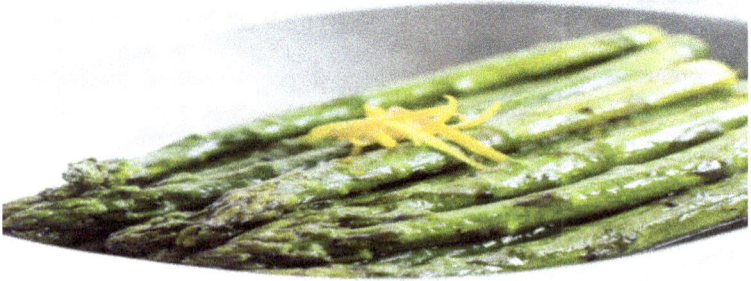

Lemon juice is rich in essential nutrients — such as vitamin A, vitamin C, folate, calcium, magnesium, phosphorous, and potassium — and is a good source of healthy sugars for those sweet recipes you crave. Yet, lemon juice has also been found to have anti-fungal properties, as well as "help detoxify your liver," both of which aid the body heal and fight fungal infections. This recipe calls for lemon zest — shavings of lemon rind — balancing out the sweetness of the juice, as well as healthy fat-rich olive oil.

11. Blood Orange, Carrot and Ginger Smoothie

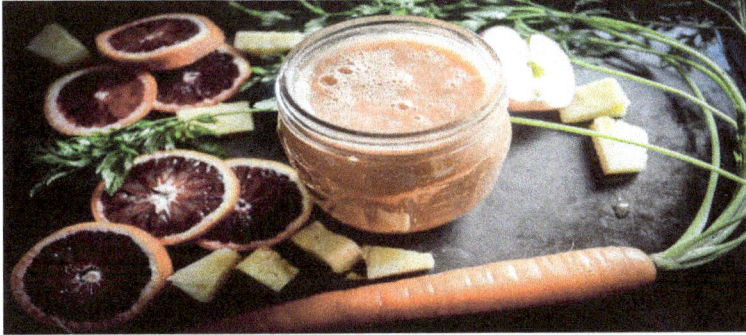

Smoothies are an excellent way to get your necessary dose of essential nutrients without a kitchen handy. This Blood Orange, Carrot and Ginger Smoothie has the added benefit of using fungus-fighting coconut milk and grated fresh ginger. Plus, the powerful mixture of antioxidants and vitamin C from the carrots and pineapple, the pectin (a unique form of fiber) from apples, and the inflammation-fighting and folic acid rich blood orange, make this the perfect smoothie to fight off ailments of any kind or simply keep a healthy body healthy!

12. Chaga Vinegar

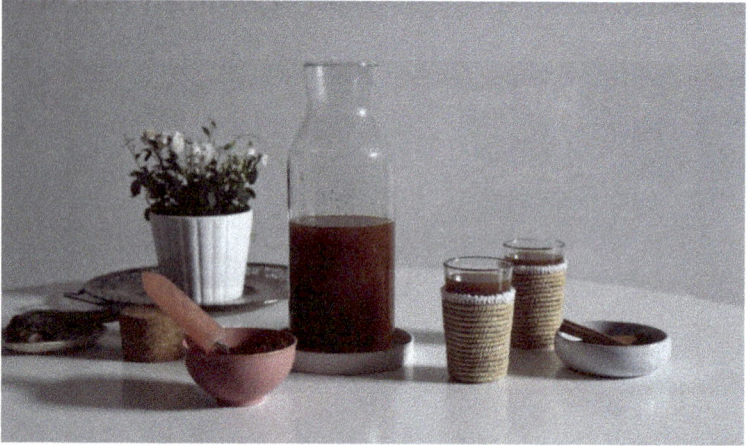

This Chaga Vinegar only has four simple ingredients: A third of a cup of adaptogenic Chaga mushrooms will help level out your body's natural stress response, lower anxiety, and provide energy. A full liter of apple cider, plus a cinnamon stick will fight fungal infections and provide a detoxifying effect. Plus, that vanilla bean has health benefits as well such as fighting acne, reducing anxiety, and promoting good digestion!

13. Patatas Bravas with Garlic Aioli

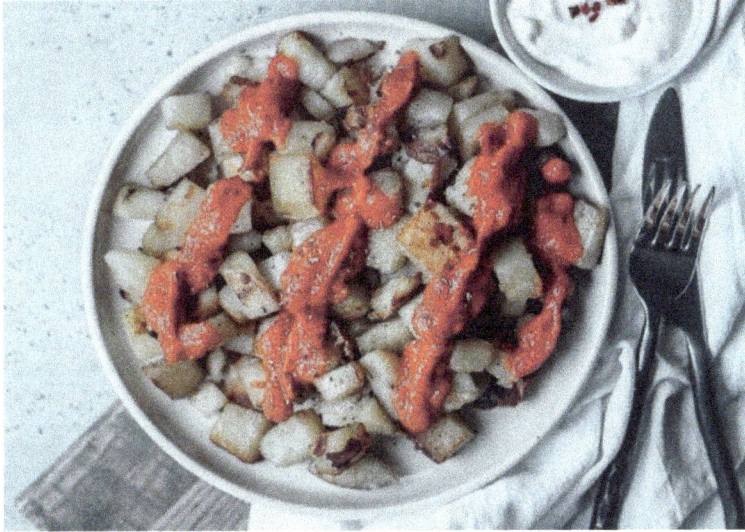

This dairy-free, vegan Patatas Bravas with Garlic Aioli recipe is a great way to get your daily dose of fungus-fighting garlic, as well as a slew of other nutrient-rich, plant-based food. This patatas bravas call for around four minced cloves of garlic, as well as fungus-fighting onions, and healthy fat-rich olive oil!

14. Coconut Oil Cookies

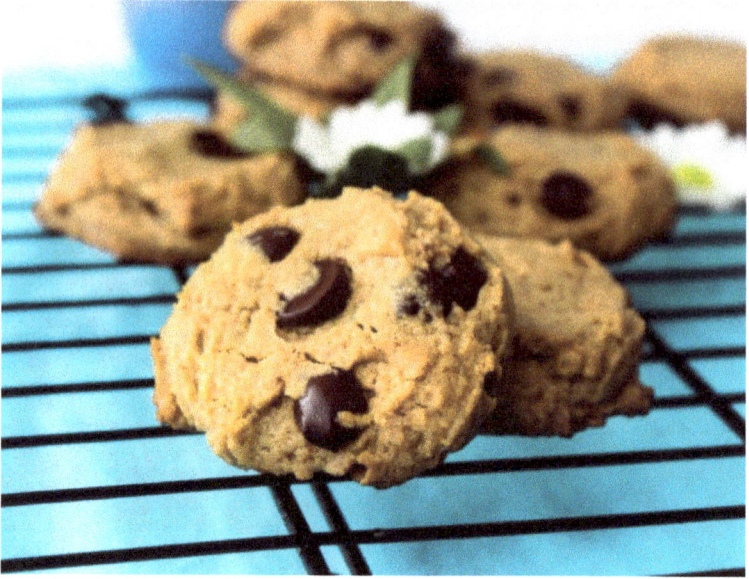

Hankering for something sweet? Instead of reaching for that pre-packaged box of cookies — filled with processed ingredients — try having these Coconut Oil Cookies on hand! They are rich in fungus-fighting coconut oil, nutrient-filled coconut sugar, and fiber-filled nuts!

15. Onion and Pepper Masala

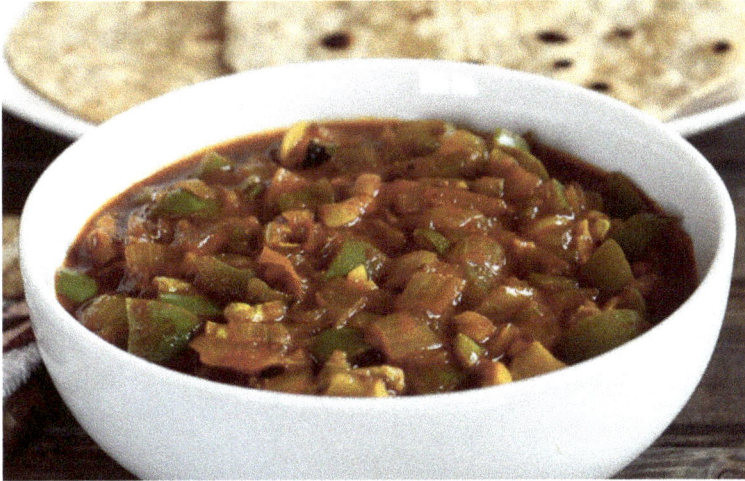

Onions are a great side addition to meals that require a bit more flavor, yet they can also be the main player! This Onion and Pepper not only favors onions — one large onion, in fact — but it also incorporates other fungus-fighting agents such as cloves, ginger, and oil of your choice (substitute coconut oil!). Plus, it incorporates other anti-inflammatory foods such as turmeric — rich in curcumin — and antioxidant-rich bell peppers.

www.ingramcontent.com/pod-product-compliance
Lightning Source LLC
Chambersburg PA
CBHW071514210326
41597CB00018B/2748